Funny Feelings Aren't Funny

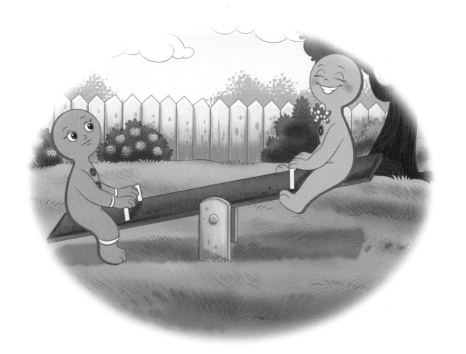

Kim May

Illustrated by Anisha Singha

Typesetting and layout: WorkingType www.workingtype.com.au

Published January 2019

For all our children

Funny feelings, they aren't funny,

Funny feelings, they aren't great,

Funny feelings, I don't feel safe,

So help me to communicate.

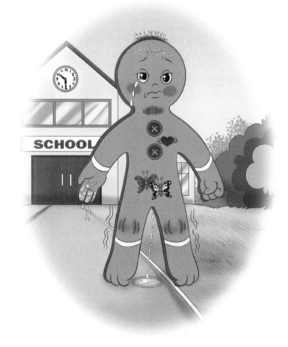

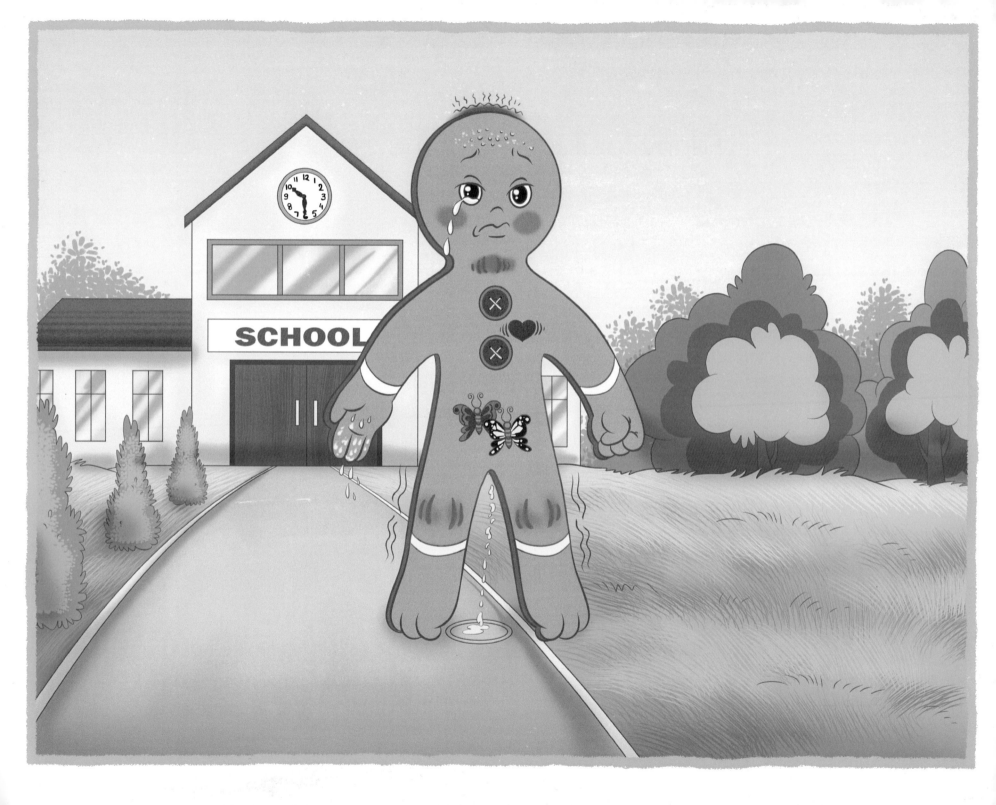

Funny feelings make me sweat,

It's not hot,

But my face is wet.

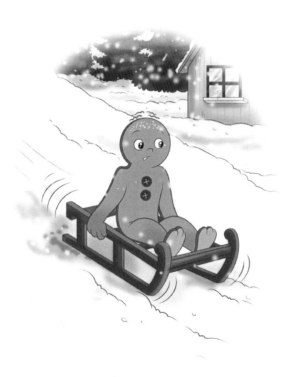

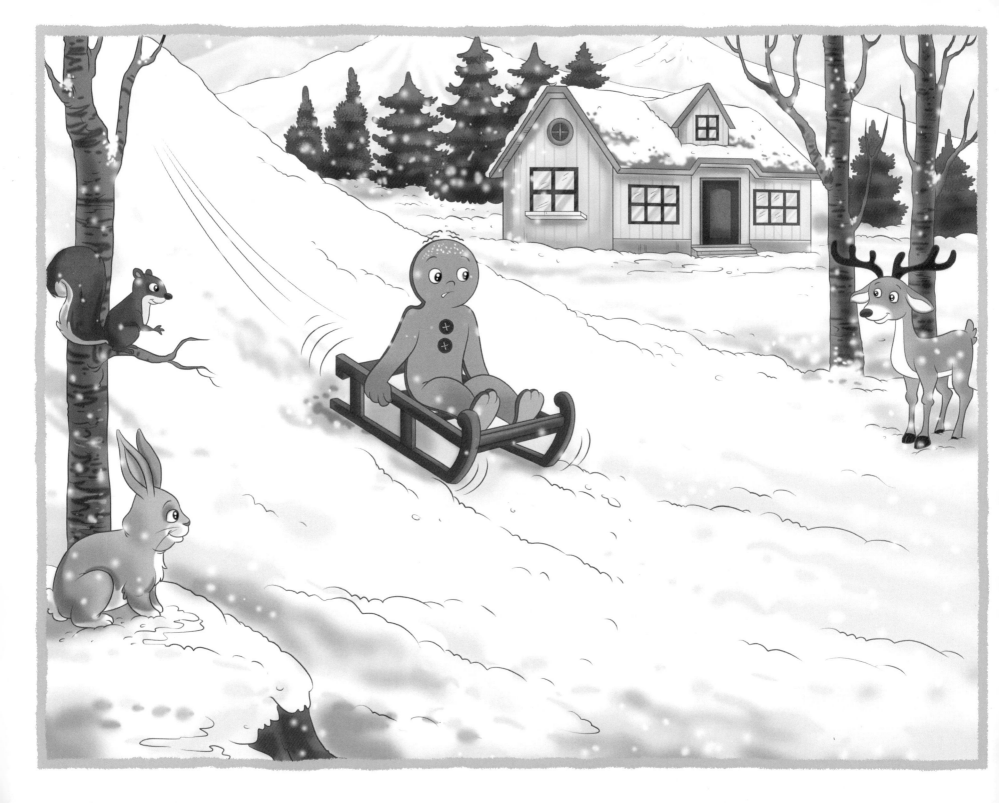

Funny feelings,

Thump, thump, thump,

Pounding heart,

Makes me jump.

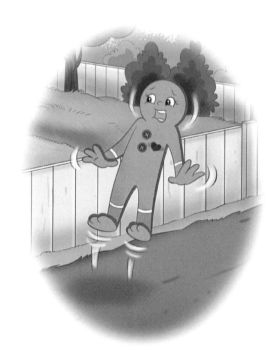

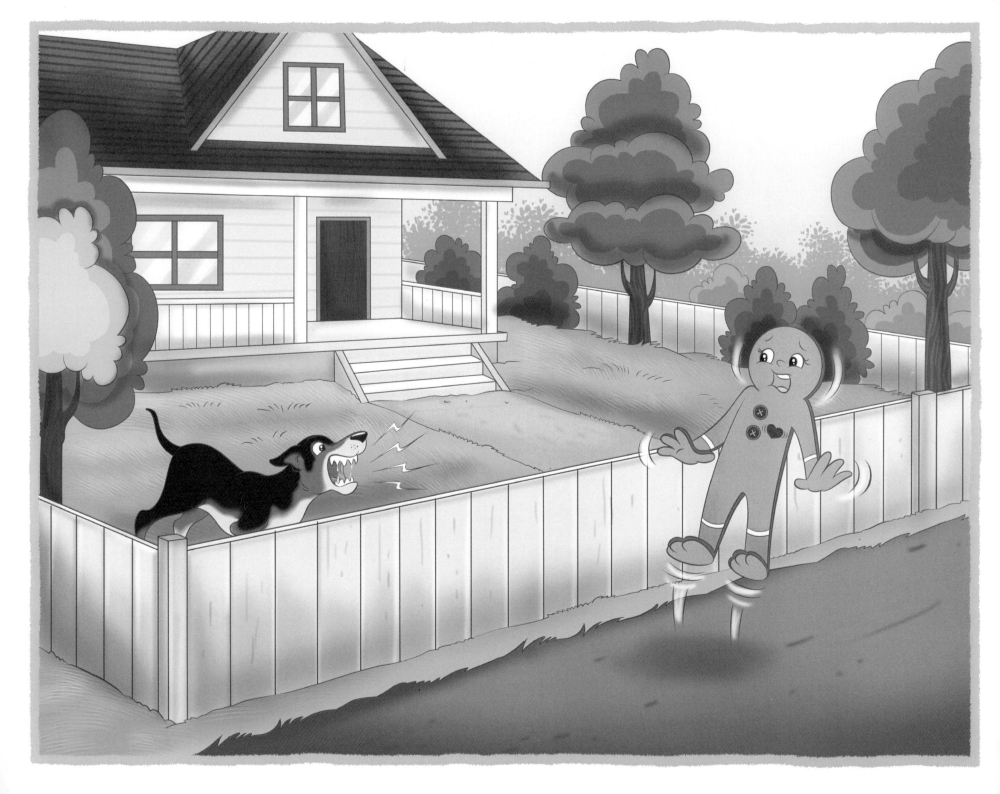

Funny feelings in my head,
Goodness gracious,
My cheeks are red.

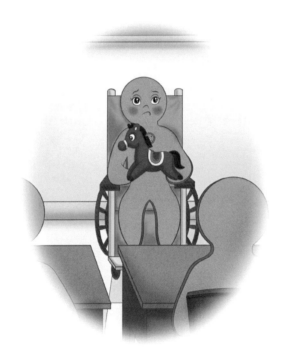

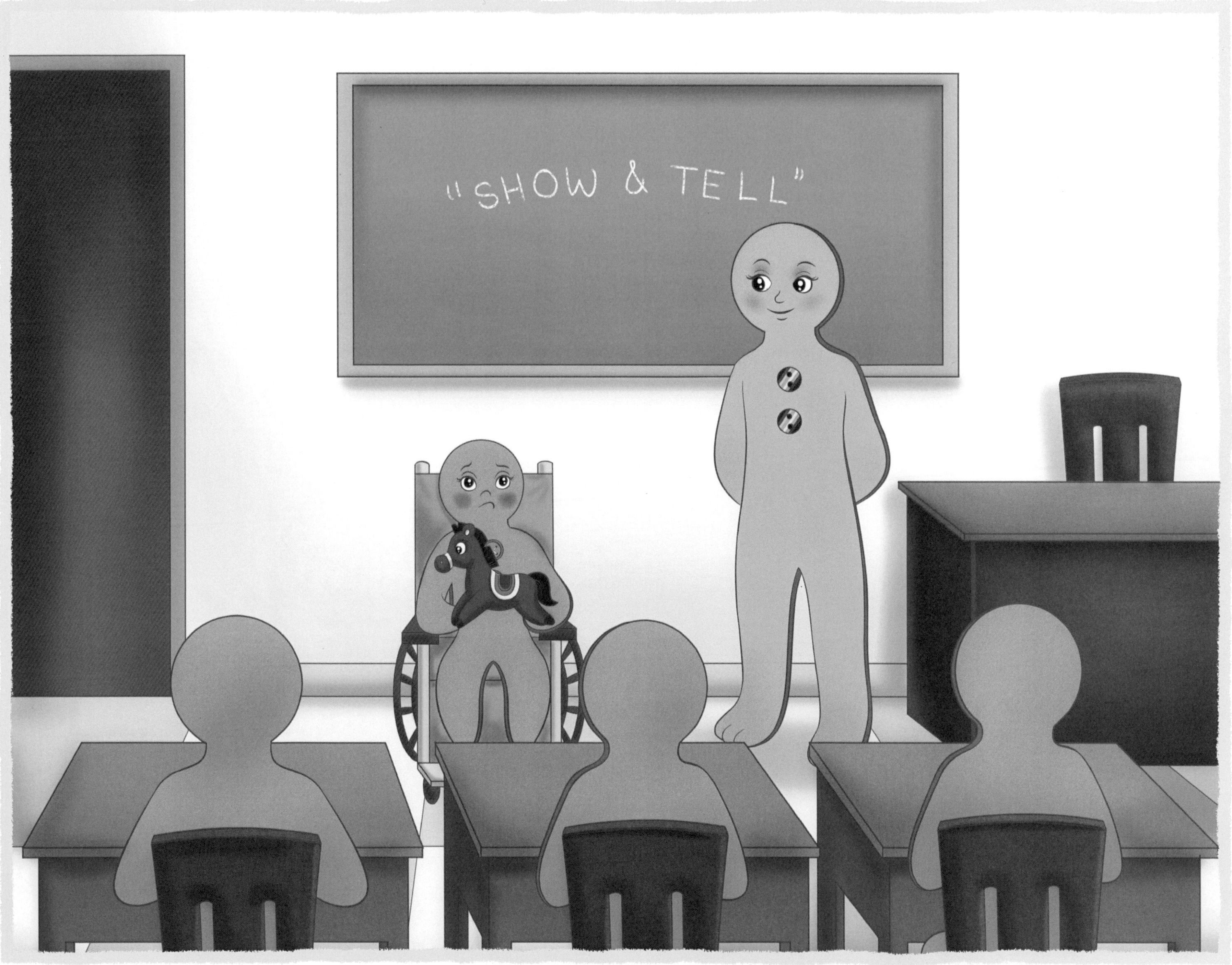
"SHOW & TELL"

Funny feelings, something is stuck,

No, nothing is there,

It just feels yuck.

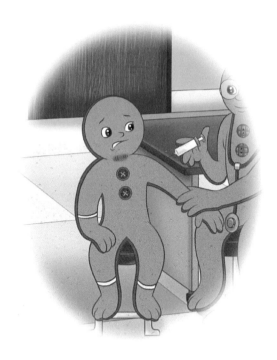

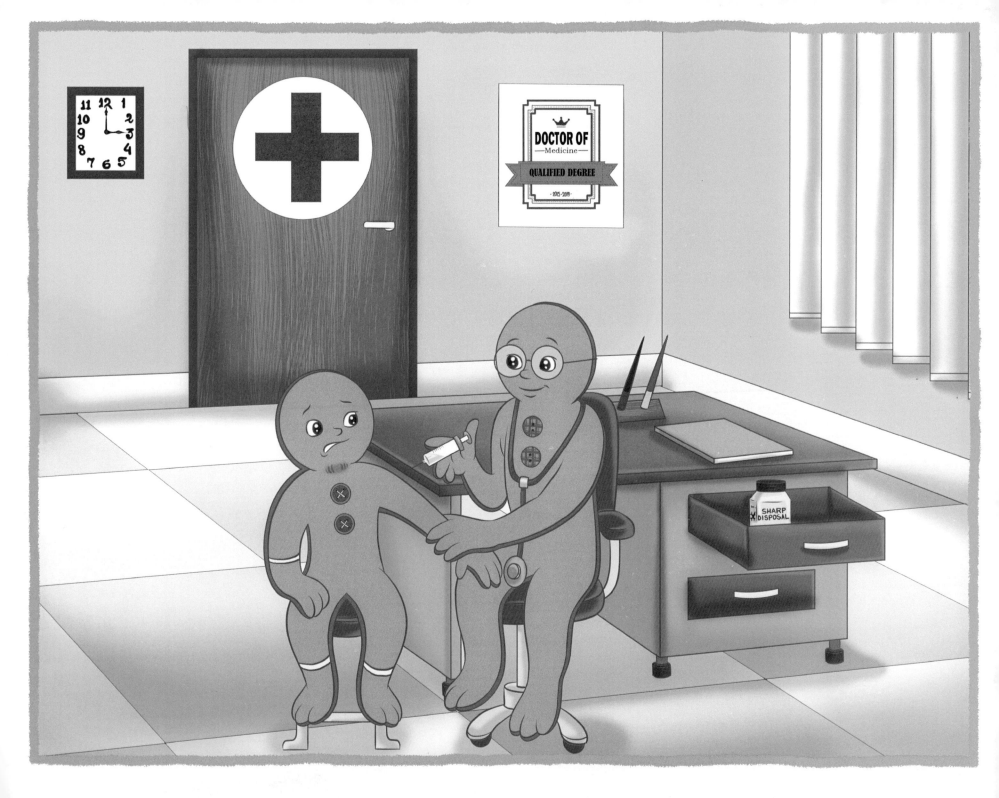

Funny feelings in my tummy,

Funny feelings sure aren't funny.

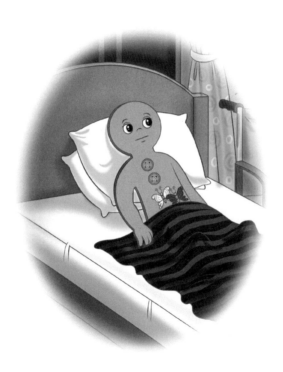

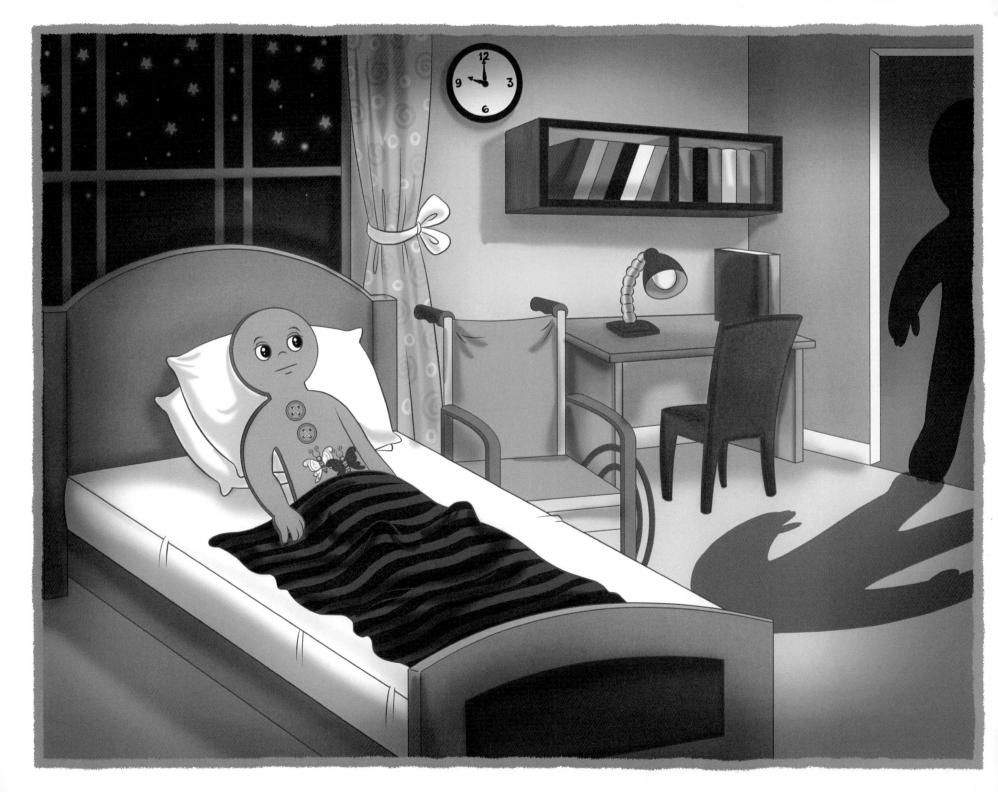

Funny feelings,

Wobbly knees,

I can't stop shaking,

So help me please.

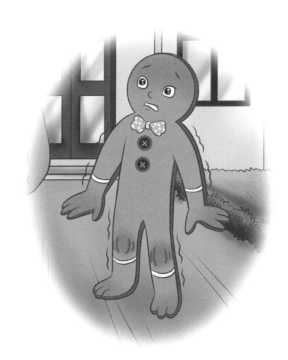

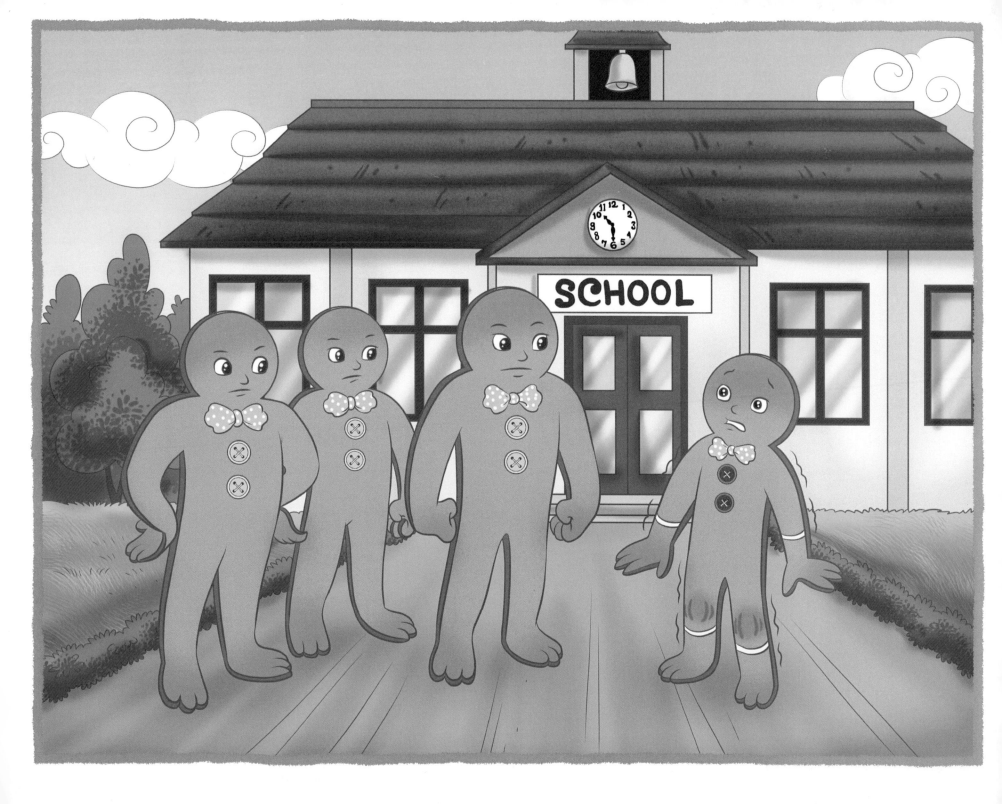

Funny feelings,
I don't like what I see,
I run to the bathroom,
Before I pee.

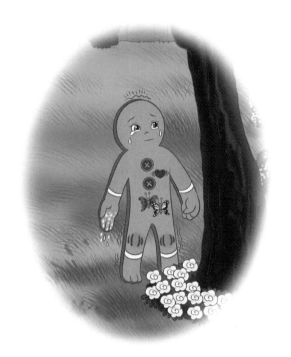

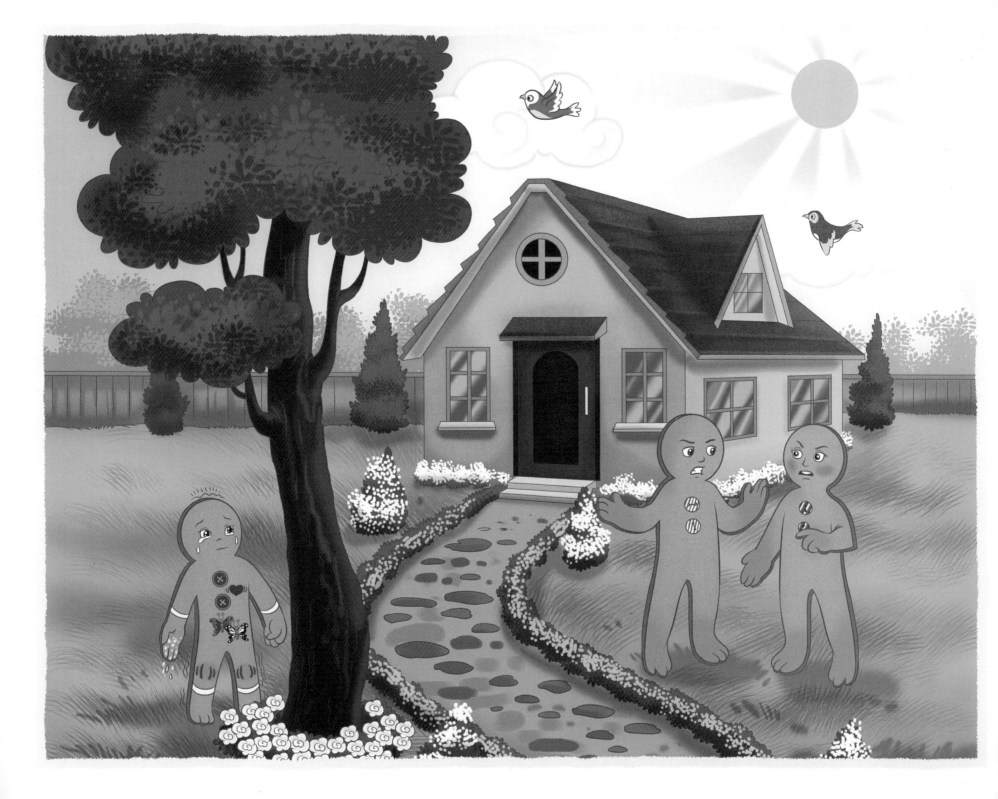

Funny feelings,
Tears in my eyes,
I'm not sad,
But I want to cry.

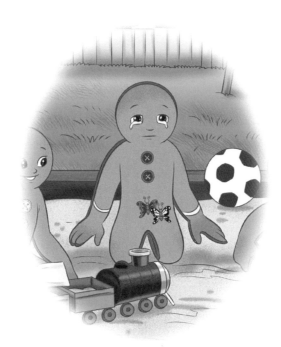

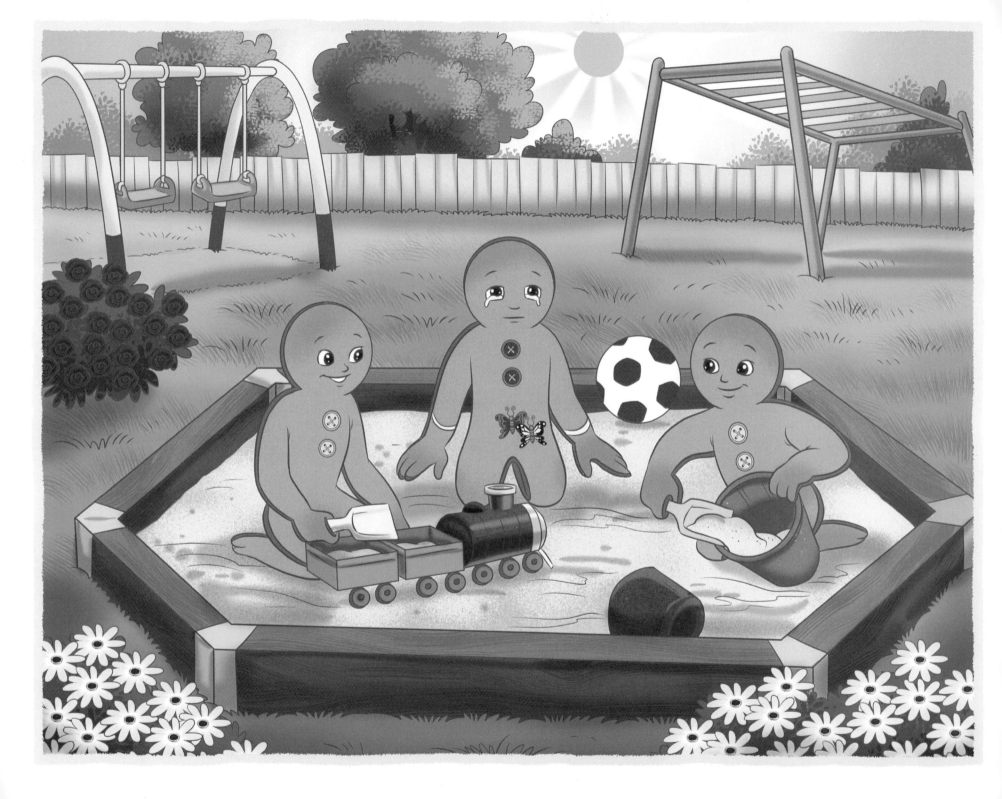

Funny feelings, when I just know,

There are places I don't want to go.

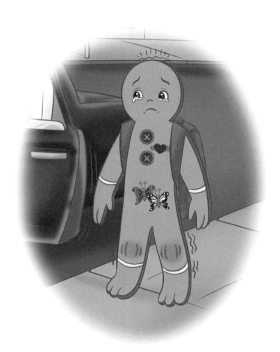

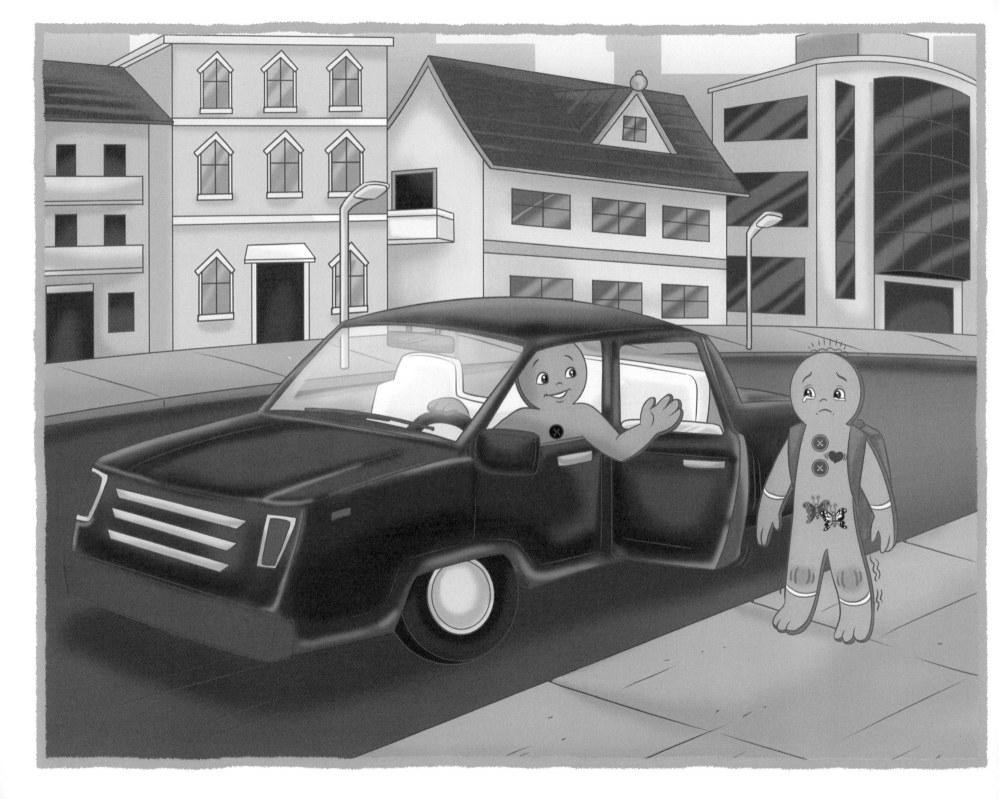

Funny feelings, day or night,

Maybe something is not quite right?

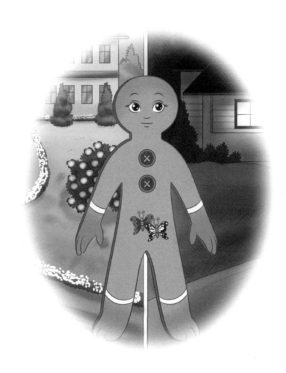

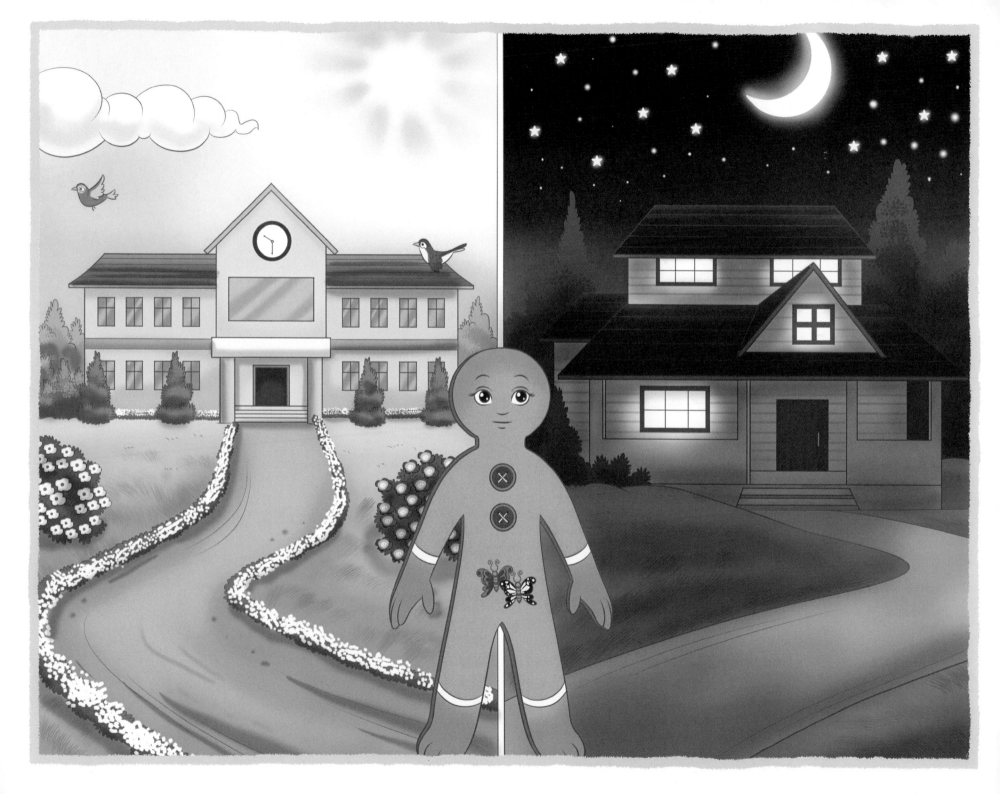

Funny feelings, help me please,

To tell someone what they cannot see.

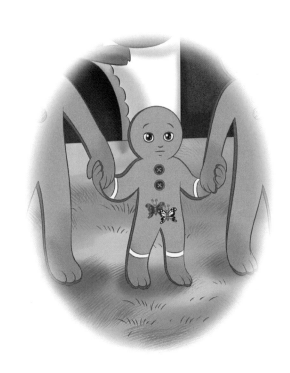

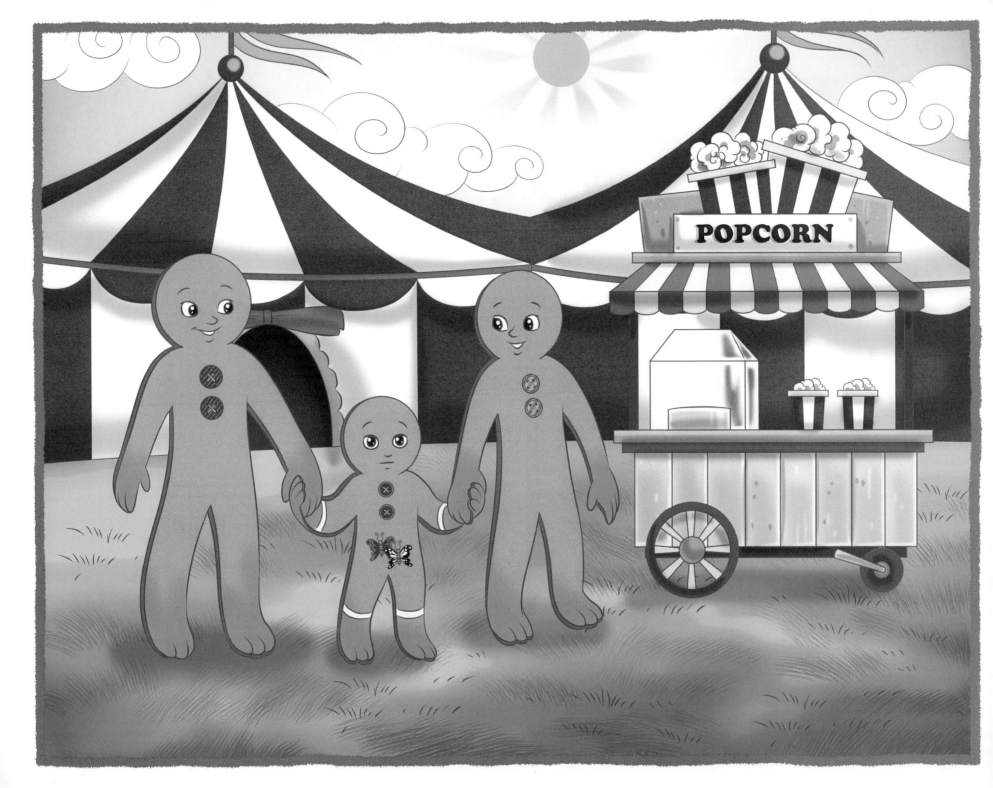

Funny feelings, I must share,

With someone who I know will care.

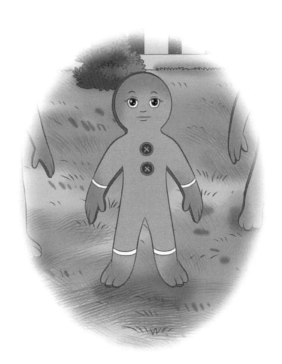

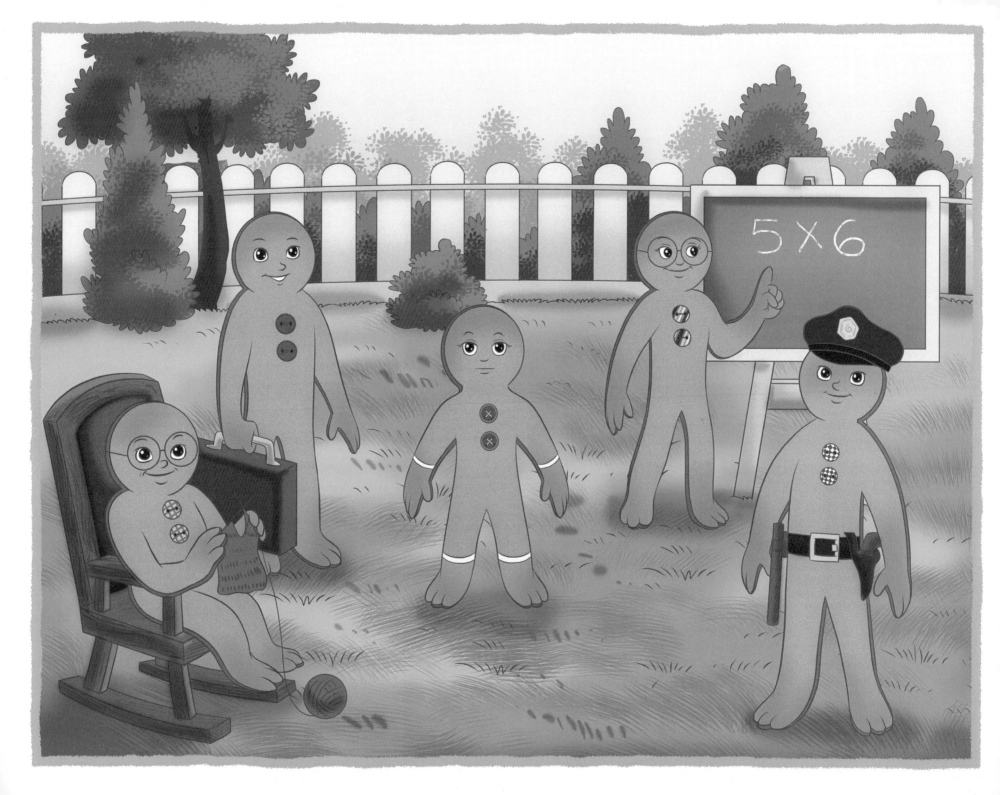

Funny feelings, they aren't funny,

Funny feelings, they aren't great,

Funny feelings, I told someone,

YOU helped me to communicate!

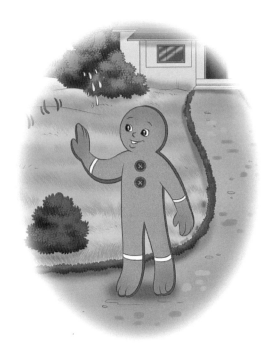

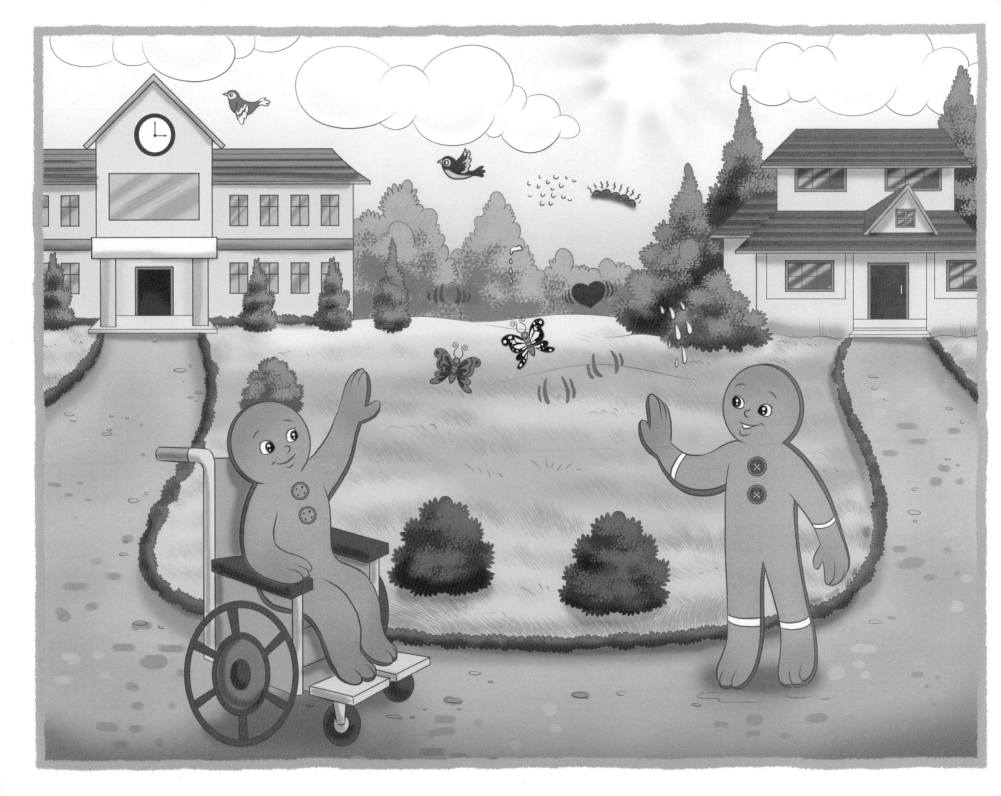

Lightning Source UK Ltd.
Milton Keynes UK
UKRC011511240920
370393UK00003B/5

9 780648 474005